Kegel Exercise And Workouts Guide

A Complete Step-by-Step Guide to Doing Kegel Exercises Correctly Boosting Strength Gains Twice

Vicky Klocko

Table of Contents

CHAPTER ONE

Introduction

Kegel exercises are great for strengthening pelvic floor muscles. To get started, identify the muscles by stopping the flow of urine midstream (do this only to identify, not during actual exercises). Then, empty your bladder and lie down. Contract these muscles for 5 seconds, then relax for 5 seconds. Aim for 3 sets of 10 repetitions a day. Incorporating a camera snapping feature could be a reminder to do these exercises regularly, like a visual cue on your phone or a wearable device. Would

CHAPTER ONE
Introduction

Kegel exercises are great for strengthening pelvic floor muscles. To get started, identify the muscles by stopping the flow of urine midstream (do this only to identify, not during actual exercises). Then, empty your bladder and lie down. Contract these muscles for 5 seconds, then relax for 5 seconds. Aim for 3 sets of 10 repetitions a day. Incorporating a camera snapping feature could be a reminder to do these exercises regularly, like a visual cue on your phone or a wearable device. Would you like more details or specific exercises?

What is a Kegel exercise?

Kegel exercises involve contracting and relaxing the pelvic floor muscles. These muscles support the bladder, uterus, rectum, and small intestine. The exercises aim to strengthen these muscles, which can help with bladder control, especially for individuals experiencing urinary incontinence. They're also beneficial for sexual function by potentially enhancing sensation and improving orgasms. The exercises are usually done by squeezing the pelvic floor muscles, holding for a few seconds, and then releasing.

Needs for kegel exercise

Kegel exercises are helpful for various reasons:

Urinary Incontinence: Strengthening the pelvic floor muscles can help prevent or reduce leakage of urine, especially when coughing, laughing, sneezing, or exercising.

Postpartum Recovery: After childbirth, these exercises can aid in restoring pelvic muscle strength, potentially reducing bladder control problems.

Improved Sexual Health: Stronger pelvic floor muscles can enhance sexual pleasure and improve orgasm control for both men and women.

Preventing Prolapse: Strengthening these muscles may help prevent pelvic organs from sagging or dropping, known as pelvic organ prolapse.

Preparation for Surgery: For individuals undergoing prostate surgery or hysterectomy, pre-surgery and post-surgery exercises can aid in a faster recovery.

What do Kegel exercises actually do?

Kegel exercises primarily target and strengthen the pelvic floor muscles. These muscles play a crucial role in supporting the pelvic organs, including the bladder, uterus, rectum, and small intestine. Strengthening these muscles through Kegel exercises can have several benefits:

Improving Bladder Control: Stronger pelvic floor muscles can help prevent or reduce urinary incontinence, particularly stress incontinence, where urine leaks during activities like coughing, sneezing, or exercising.

Enhancing Sexual Function: For both men and women, stronger pelvic floor muscles can lead to improved sexual function. For men, it can potentially help with erectile dysfunction, while for women, it may increase sensation and improve orgasm intensity.

Aiding in Postpartum Recovery: After childbirth, these exercises can help restore pelvic muscle strength, reducing the risk of urinary incontinence and supporting faster recovery of pelvic muscles.

Supporting Pelvic Organ Health: Strengthening these muscles may help prevent pelvic organ prolapse, where organs like the bladder, uterus, or rectum descend into the vagina due to weak pelvic floor muscles.

Preparation for Certain Surgeries: Pre-surgery and post-surgery Kegel exercises are often recommended for individuals undergoing procedures like prostate surgery or hysterectomy to aid in recovery.

Overall, Kegel exercises are simple yet effective in improving pelvic floor muscle strength, which can positively impact various aspects of urinary, sexual, and pelvic health.

Peoples who needs to do Kegels

Kegel exercises can benefit various groups of people:

Women: Especially those who are pregnant or have recently given birth. Pregnancy and childbirth can weaken pelvic floor muscles, leading to urinary incontinence. Kegels can help prevent or alleviate this.

Men and Women with Urinary Incontinence: Individuals experiencing leakage during activities like coughing, sneezing, or exercising may find Kegel exercises helpful in improving bladder control.

Men: Particularly those dealing with urinary incontinence after prostate surgery or seeking to improve erectile dysfunction. Kegels can strengthen the pelvic floor muscles, potentially aiding in these issues.

Those with Pelvic Organ Prolapse: Strengthening the pelvic floor muscles may help prevent or alleviate pelvic organ prolapse, where pelvic organs drop due to weak support.

People Seeking Sexual Health Benefits: Both men and women can benefit from improved sexual function, potentially enhancing sensation and orgasm control.

Essentially, anyone looking to strengthen their pelvic floor muscles or experiencing issues related to bladder control, postpartum recovery, or sexual function could consider incorporating Kegel exercises into their routine.

CHAPTER TWO

Types of kegel exercise

There are various types of Kegel exercises that target the pelvic floor muscles. Here are a few:

Standard Kegels: These involve contracting the pelvic floor muscles and holding for a few seconds before releasing. Start with 5-second holds and gradually work up to 10 seconds or more.

Quick Flicks: Rapidly contract and relax the pelvic floor muscles. This exercise focuses on building muscle endurance.

Elevator Kegels: Gradually tighten the pelvic floor muscles, as if you're moving up floors in an elevator. Start with a slight contraction and gradually increase the intensity until you've contracted as strongly as possible. Then, gradually release, as if descending floors.

Bridge or Modified Squats: These exercises incorporate movements like bridges or modified squats to engage the pelvic floor muscles along with other muscle groups.

Biofeedback-Assisted Kegels: Some devices or apps provide biofeedback to help you identify and strengthen the correct muscles by providing visual or auditory cues.

Remember, it's important to identify the right muscles first. Imagine stopping the flow of urine or tightening the muscles used to prevent passing gas. Once you've identified them, incorporate these different types of exercises into your routine to target and strengthen the pelvic floor muscles effectively. Starting with the basic holds and gradually progressing to other variations can be a good approach.

Benefits of kegel exercise

Kegel exercises offer a range of benefits, primarily focusing on strengthening the pelvic floor muscles. Some of the key benefits include:

Improved Bladder Control: Strengthening these muscles can help prevent or reduce urinary incontinence, especially stress incontinence, where urine leaks during activities like coughing, laughing, or exercising.

Enhanced Sexual Function: Both men and women may experience improved sexual health. For men, stronger pelvic floor muscles can assist with erectile dysfunction, while for women, it may increase sensation and lead to more intense orgasms.

Postpartum Recovery: After childbirth, Kegel exercises can aid in restoring pelvic muscle strength, reducing the risk of urinary incontinence and supporting faster recovery.

Support for Pelvic Organ Health: Strengthening these muscles may help prevent pelvic organ prolapse, where pelvic organs descend due to weak support.

Preparation for Surgery: Pre-surgery and post-surgery Kegel exercises are often recommended for individuals undergoing procedures like prostate surgery or hysterectomy to aid in recovery.

Enhanced Confidence: Improving bladder control and sexual function can contribute to increased confidence and overall well-being.

Regularly practicing Kegel exercises can significantly benefit pelvic health, urinary control, sexual satisfaction, and overall quality of life.

Methods of performing kegel exercise

Performing Kegel exercises involves identifying and contracting the pelvic floor muscles. Here's a step-by-step guide:

Identify the Muscles:

To identify the right muscles, try stopping the flow of urine midstream. However, don't regularly practice Kegels while urinating, as it may cause bladder issues.

Another method is to tighten the muscles used to prevent passing gas. These are the same muscles targeted in Kegel exercises.

Find a Comfortable Position:

You can perform Kegels in various positions: lying down, sitting, or standing. Choose the one that's most comfortable for you.

Perform the Exercises:

Contract the pelvic floor muscles. Imagine pulling them up and in.

Hold the contraction for 3-5 seconds when starting. Gradually increase to 10 seconds as you gain strength.

Relax the muscles for an equal amount of time as you contracted them.

Repeat Regularly:

Aim for 3 sets of 10 repetitions per day.

It's essential to be consistent for these exercises to be effective.

Avoid Tension in Other Muscles:

Ensure that you're not tightening your abdomen, buttocks, or thighs. Focus solely on the pelvic floor muscles.

Breathe Normally:

Maintain regular breathing throughout the exercise; avoid holding your breath.

Gradually Increase Intensity:

As you gain strength, you can increase the duration of contractions and the number of repetitions.

Use Visual or Auditory Cues:

Some apps or devices provide biofeedback, helping you identify and strengthen the correct muscles by providing visual or auditory cues.

Consistency is key with Kegel exercises. Incorporating them into your daily routine can gradually strengthen the pelvic floor muscles, leading to various health benefits.

CHAPTER THREE

Pregnancy and Kegel exercises

Kegel exercises can be particularly beneficial during pregnancy and after childbirth:

During Pregnancy:

Strengthening the pelvic floor muscles can help prepare the body for childbirth.

Kegel exercises can assist in maintaining bladder control during pregnancy when the growing baby puts pressure on the bladder.

Improved pelvic muscle strength can aid in postpartum recovery.

Postpartum Recovery:

After childbirth, pelvic floor muscles can be weakened due to the strain of pregnancy and delivery.

Kegel exercises can help restore pelvic muscle strength, potentially reducing the risk of urinary incontinence and supporting faster recovery.

It's essential for pregnant women to perform Kegel exercises correctly and regularly, but it's equally important to consult a healthcare provider before starting any new exercise regimen during pregnancy. They can provide guidance on the appropriate timing, frequency, and technique to ensure safety and effectiveness. In some cases, they might recommend avoiding certain exercises during pregnancy, especially if there are specific medical concerns.

To find my pelvic floor muscles

Locating your pelvic floor muscles can be done through a few different methods:

Stop Urine Flow: While urinating, try to stop the flow of urine midstream. The muscles you use to do this are your pelvic floor muscles. However, it's important not to make a habit of regularly doing Kegel exercises while urinating, as it can disrupt normal bladder emptying.

Imagine Holding Gas: Another way to locate these muscles is by imagining you're trying to hold in gas. The muscles you engage to prevent passing gas are the same ones involved in Kegel exercises.

Importance Of Kegel exercises

Kegel exercises matter for several important reasons:

Bladder Control: Strengthening the pelvic floor muscles can significantly improve bladder control, reducing or preventing urinary incontinence, especially stress incontinence.

Postpartum Recovery: After childbirth, these exercises help in restoring pelvic muscle strength, aiding in the recovery process and potentially reducing the risk of urinary incontinence.

Sexual Health: Strong pelvic floor muscles can enhance sexual function, leading to increased sensation and potentially more intense orgasms for both men and women.

Preventing Pelvic Organ Prolapse: Strengthening these muscles may prevent or alleviate pelvic organ prolapse, where pelvic organs sag or drop due to weak support.

Support for Surgery: Pre-surgery and post-surgery Kegel exercises are often recommended for individuals undergoing procedures like prostate surgery or hysterectomy to aid in recovery.

Confidence and Well-being:
Improved bladder control and sexual function contribute to increased confidence and overall well-being.

Regularly practicing Kegel exercises can significantly benefit pelvic health, urinary control, sexual satisfaction, and overall quality of life. These exercises are simple yet impactful in maintaining and improving various aspects of health and well-being.

Methods to do Kegel exercises

Performing Kegel exercises involves a few straightforward steps:

Identify the Muscles:

To locate the right muscles, try to stop the flow of urine midstream. However, avoid frequently doing Kegels while urinating as it can disrupt bladder function.

Another method is to tighten the muscles you use to prevent passing gas. These are the same muscles targeted in Kegel exercises.

Find a Comfortable Position:

You can perform Kegels while lying down, sitting, or standing. Choose the position that's most comfortable for you.

Perform the Exercises:

Contract the pelvic floor muscles by squeezing or pulling them inward and upward.

Hold the contraction for 3-5 seconds initially. Gradually work up to holding for 10 seconds as you gain strength.

Release and relax the muscles for an equal amount of time as you contracted them.

Repeat Regularly:

Aim for 3 sets of 10 repetitions per day.

Consistency is key for Kegel exercises to be effective.

Focus and Relax:

Ensure you're only tightening the pelvic floor muscles without engaging other muscles like the abdomen, buttocks, or thighs.

Breathe normally during the exercises; avoid holding your breath.

Gradually Increase Intensity:

As your strength improves, you can increase the duration of contractions and the number of repetitions.

Use Visual or Auditory Cues:

Apps or devices can provide biofeedback to help identify and strengthen the correct muscles by offering visual or auditory cues.

Remember, it's essential to do Kegel exercises correctly and consistently to effectively strengthen the pelvic floor muscles.

CHAPTER FOUR

When to Perform Kegels

You can do Kegel exercises at any time that fits your schedule, but here are some suggestions on when to incorporate them:

Regular Routine: Establish a routine where you perform Kegels at the same time every day. This consistency helps in forming a habit.

During Daily Activities: Incorporate Kegel exercises while performing daily tasks like sitting at your desk, watching TV, or waiting in line. These moments can serve as reminders to do your exercises.

Posture Change: Some people find it helpful to do Kegels when changing positions, such as moving from sitting to standing or vice versa.

Before and After Specific Activities: Consider doing Kegels before and after activities that might put stress on your pelvic floor muscles, like lifting heavy objects or exercising.

Natural Cues: Use natural cues like waiting for a red light while driving, brushing your teeth, or during specific

breaks in your daily routine.

Problems In doing Kegel Exercises

If you're having trouble performing

Kegel exercises or experiencing

difficulties, here are some suggestions

to help:

Proper Identification: Ensure you're

targeting the correct muscles. Try

different methods to locate your pelvic

floor muscles, such as stopping urine

flow or imagining holding in gas.

Relaxed Environment: Find a quiet, comfortable place where you can focus without distractions.

Practice Regularly: Consistency is crucial. Set a routine and try to perform Kegels at the same time every day.

Visual or Auditory Cues: Use apps or devices that provide biofeedback to help identify and strengthen the correct muscles by offering visual or auditory cues.

Seek Professional Guidance: If you're unsure about the technique or having difficulties, consult a healthcare professional, such as a doctor, physical therapist, or pelvic health specialist. They can provide personalized guidance and exercises tailored to your needs.

Patience and Persistence: It may take time to notice improvements. Be patient and persistent in practicing Kegel exercises regularly.

Remember, it's normal to encounter challenges when starting any new exercise routine. With practice and guidance, you can improve your ability to perform Kegel exercises effectively.

Results Expectations In kegel Exercises

The timeline for seeing results from Kegel exercises can vary from person to person. Factors such as consistency, starting muscle strength, and individual differences can influence how soon you notice improvements. Generally:

Initial Sensation: Some people may notice a difference in sensation or muscle awareness within a few weeks of starting Kegel exercises. This might include feeling more in control of the pelvic muscles or a slight improvement in bladder control.

Noticeable Improvements: Significant improvements in bladder control or pelvic muscle strength might take several weeks to a few months of consistent practice.

Long-Term Benefits: Continuously practicing Kegel exercises over time can lead to lasting improvements in bladder control, pelvic muscle strength, and even sexual satisfaction.

It's essential to be patient and consistent with Kegel exercises.

Ways To Know You Are Doing Kegels Exercises correctly

Ensuring you're doing Kegel exercises correctly involves a few indicators:

Sensation of Contraction: You should feel a tightening or squeezing sensation in the pelvic floor muscles without engaging other muscle groups like the abdomen, buttocks, or thighs.

No Straining or Holding Breath: Proper Kegel exercises should not involve straining, and you should be able to continue regular breathing throughout the exercise.

Pelvic Movement: There shouldn't be any noticeable movement in your pelvis, abdomen, or legs while performing Kegels. The movement should be isolated to the pelvic floor muscles.

Consistency of Practice: Regular practice with consistent improvement over time is a good indicator that you're doing Kegels correctly. Over weeks or months, you might notice improved bladder control or pelvic muscle strength.

Seeking Professional Guidance: If you're unsure whether you're doing

Kegel exercises correctly, consulting a healthcare professional, such as a doctor or physical therapist, can provide guidance. They might use techniques like biofeedback to confirm if you're engaging the correct muscles.

CHAPTER FIVE

How To know if my pelvic floor is strong

Determining the strength of your pelvic floor muscles can involve various indicators:

Urinary Control: Strong pelvic floor muscles can contribute to better control over urinary functions. If you experience fewer incidents of urine leakage or improved ability to hold urine when needed, it might indicate stronger pelvic floor muscles.

Sensations during Kegels: When performing Kegel exercises, a sense of control and the ability to contract and relax these muscles effectively can indicate strength.

Sustained Contractions: Strong pelvic floor muscles can maintain contractions for longer durations without fatigue or difficulty.

Pelvic Organ Support: Strong pelvic floor muscles might contribute to better support for pelvic organs, potentially reducing the risk of pelvic organ prolapse.

How hard To squeeze for Kegels

The intensity of the squeeze during Kegel exercises should be enough to engage and contract the pelvic floor muscles without causing discomfort or straining other muscle groups. It's essential to find a balance:

Start Gradually: Begin with a gentle contraction, gradually increasing the intensity as you become more accustomed to the exercises.

Sufficient but Comfortable: The squeeze should be strong enough to feel the muscles working without causing pain, discomfort, or straining other muscles like the abdomen or buttocks.

Avoid Overexertion: Avoid excessively tight or forceful contractions as they might lead to muscle fatigue or tension.

Focus on Control: Focus on the quality of the contraction rather than the intensity. Aim for a controlled and steady contraction and release.

Consistency is Key: Regular practice and consistency are more important than extreme force. Building muscle strength over time is the goal.

Better Way To Do Kegels Exercises (sitting or standing)

Both sitting and standing positions can be effective for doing Kegel exercises. The key is to choose a position where you can easily identify and isolate the pelvic floor muscles and perform the exercises comfortably. Here's a comparison:

Sitting:

Many find it easier to concentrate and focus on the pelvic floor muscles while sitting.

Sitting might offer better relaxation of surrounding muscles, allowing for better isolation of the targeted muscles.

It can be more comfortable for some individuals, especially when starting the exercises.

Standing:

Standing can engage additional muscles for stability and balance, which might make it slightly more challenging to isolate the pelvic floor muscles.

Some people find it easier to incorporate Kegel exercises into their daily routine while standing, such as during a commute or while waiting in line.Ultimately, the best position for doing Kegel exercises is the one that allows you to properly identify and contract the pelvic floor muscles without straining other muscle groups. Experiment with both positions to determine which works best for you in terms of comfort, concentration, and ease of practice.

Durations To hold A Kegel

When starting Kegel exercises, begin by holding the contraction for a few seconds and gradually increase the duration as your pelvic floor muscles strengthen. Here's a general guideline:

Start with 3-5 Seconds: When initiating Kegel exercises, aim to hold the contraction for about 3-5 seconds initially. This duration allows you to focus on engaging the muscles without straining.

Gradually Increase: As your muscles become stronger, gradually extend the duration of the holds. Work towards holding the contraction for 10 seconds or more, aiming for a sustained and controlled contraction without causing discomfort.

Focus on Quality: Focus on the quality of the contraction rather than holding for an excessively long time. It's crucial to maintain a controlled and steady contraction throughout the hold.

Consistency is Key: Consistently practicing Kegel exercises at a duration that challenges your muscles without causing strain or discomfort is more important than aiming for a specific number of seconds initially.

Best Kegel exercise

The "best" Kegel exercise can vary based on individual preferences and needs. However, some effective variations include:

Standard Kegels: Contracting and holding the pelvic floor muscles for a few seconds before releasing. It's a foundational exercise for strengthening these muscles.

Quick Flicks: Rapidly contracting and relaxing the pelvic floor muscles. This exercise focuses on building muscle endurance.

Elevator Kegels: Gradually tightening the pelvic floor muscles from a gentle contraction to a strong hold, then gradually releasing, mimicking an elevator moving up and down floors.

Bridge or Modified Squats: Incorporating movements like bridges or modified squats to engage the pelvic floor muscles along with other muscle groups.

Biofeedback-Assisted Kegels: Using devices or apps that provide biofeedback to help identify and strengthen the correct muscles by offering visual or auditory cues.

The effectiveness of a Kegel exercise can depend on your ability to isolate and engage the pelvic floor muscles correctly. It's often beneficial to incorporate different variations into your routine to target these muscles from various angles and improve overall strength and control.

CHAPTER SIX

Difficulties In Performing Kegel Exercises

Several factors can contribute to difficulties in performing Kegel exercises:

Incorrect Muscle Identification: Difficulty in locating and isolating the correct pelvic floor muscles can make it challenging to perform Kegels effectively.

Lack of Practice or Consistency: Like any exercise, consistent practice is essential for improvement. Lack of regularity in performing Kegel exercises might lead to difficulty in engaging these muscles.

Muscle Weakness or Fatigue: Weakness in the pelvic floor muscles or fatigue due to overexertion can make it harder to sustain contractions or perform exercises correctly.

Surrounding Muscle Tension: Tension or engagement of surrounding muscles, such as the abdomen, buttocks, or thighs, can interfere with isolating the pelvic floor muscles.

Medical Conditions: Certain medical conditions or surgeries can affect pelvic floor muscle function, making it challenging to perform Kegel exercises.

Stress or Discomfort: Stress, discomfort, or pain while performing the exercises can hinder proper engagement of the muscles.

Kegel balls

Kegel balls, also known as Ben Wa balls or pelvic floor exercise balls, are small, weighted devices designed to help strengthen the pelvic floor muscles when inserted into the vagina.

These balls typically consist of one or more small weighted balls connected by a string or silicone coating. They come in various sizes and weights to accommodate different levels of pelvic floor muscle strength.

Here is how they are used:

Insertion: The user gently inserts the Kegel balls into the vagina, similar to inserting a tampon. The string or silicone coating allows for easy removal.

Muscle Contraction: Once inserted, the pelvic floor muscles naturally contract to hold the balls in place. This involuntary action helps strengthen these muscles.

Exercise: The user can perform Kegel exercises by consciously contracting and relaxing the pelvic floor muscles while the balls are inserted. This can further enhance muscle strength and control.

Kegel balls are often recommended for individuals looking to add resistance and additional challenge to their pelvic floor exercises.

Duration it take to notice changes

The time it takes to notice changes from Kegel exercises can vary widely among individuals. Several factors can influence the timeline for observing improvements:

Consistency: Regular and consistent practice is crucial. For some, improvements may be noticed within a few weeks to a couple of months with dedicated daily practice.

Starting Muscle Strength: Individuals with weaker pelvic floor muscles might notice improvements sooner compared to those with weaker muscles.

Frequency and Duration: The frequency and duration of exercises play a role. More frequent and longer-duration sessions may potentially lead to faster progress.

Individual Differences: Everyone's body responds differently to exercises. Some may notice changes sooner, while others might take longer.

Awareness of Sensation: Changes might not always be immediately noticeable. Improved awareness of muscle control or subtle changes in bladder control might be the initial signs of progress.

Patience is Key: It's essential to remain patient and consistent. In some cases, significant improvements might take several months to become noticeable.

Persons Specialized To Perform Kegel exercises

Kegel exercises aren't exclusive to women—men can also benefit significantly from incorporating these exercises into their routine.

For men, Kegel exercises involve the same process of identifying and strengthening the pelvic floor muscles. These exercises can have several benefits:

Improving Bladder Control: Strengthening the pelvic floor muscles can help reduce urinary incontinence issues in men, especially after prostate surgery or due to other causes.

Erectile Dysfunction: Some studies suggest that Kegel exercises might help improve erectile dysfunction by enhancing blood flow to the pelvic area and improving muscle tone.

Pelvic Health: Strengthening these muscles can support better overall pelvic health and potentially aid in preventing issues like pelvic pain or discomfort.

To perform Kegel exercises, men can follow similar steps to women:

Identify the Muscles: Try stopping the flow of urine midstream or tightening the muscles used to prevent passing gas. These are the pelvic floor muscles you'll be targeting.

Perform the Exercises: Contract and hold these muscles for a few seconds before releasing. Gradually increase the duration and repetitions as the muscles become stronger.

Consistency is Key: Regular and consistent practice is essential to see improvements in bladder control and pelvic muscle strength.

Conclusion

Kegel exercises are simple yet powerful exercises that benefit both men and women by targeting and strengthening the pelvic floor muscles. These exercises offer a range of advantages, including improved bladder control, enhanced sexual function, support for pelvic health, and aiding in postpartum recovery.

Performing Kegel exercises involves identifying the pelvic floor muscles and practicing regular contractions and releases. Starting with shorter holds and gradually increasing the duration and repetitions can help in strengthening these muscles effectively. Consistency and proper technique are key to experiencing the benefits of these exercises.

For individuals facing challenges or seeking guidance, consulting a healthcare professional can provide personalized advice and exercises tailored to specific needs. Whether you're starting these exercises for the first time or looking to enhance your pelvic health, incorporating Kegel exercises into your routine can significantly contribute to overall well-being and pelvic health.

THE END